SHIBARI GUIDE FOR BEGINNERS

Discovering the Art and Philosophy of
Japanese Rope Bondage through Step-by-Step
Techniques and Colorful Pictures of Each Tie

Sakura Hoshino

TABLE OF CONTENT

INTRODUCTION

Hello dear reader, I still remember the first time I encountered Shibari, a moment etched in my mind as a turning point in my journey through life and art. It was a humid summer evening in Tokyo, where the city lights danced through the windows of a minor, intimate studio tucked away in a quiet neighborhood. The air was thick with anticipation and the soft murmur of conversation, a room filled with people who, like me, were drawn by the allure of this ancient and mysterious practice.

My journey into Shibari began as a curious observer, a seeker of understanding, wanting to explore the intricate patterns and delicate balance between freedom and restraint. As an artist and a lifelong student of human expression, I was fascinated by the possibilities that Shibari presented—an art form where the human body becomes both canvas and collaborator. It was not just about the ropes but about the stories they could tell the emotions they could evoke, and the connections they could forge.

As I stood there, watching the masterful display of rope work, I felt an undeniable pull a whisper of destiny that told me I was meant to learn this art. The ropes moved with a grace and precision that was almost hypnotic, wrapping around the model's body with a gentle yet firm embrace. It was a dance of trust and vulnerability, a silent conversation that spoke volumes without a single word. I realized then that Shibari was more than a technique; it was a language of its own, one that transcends the boundaries of culture and time.

Determined to immerse myself in this world, I sought out teachers and mentors who could guide me on this path. Each lesson was a revelation, unraveling not just the secrets of the ropes but also of myself. I learned to listen—to the subtle cues of a partner's body, to the rhythm of the ties, and to the unspoken needs that surface in the space between the knots. Shibari taught me patience and precision, respect and empathy, qualities that extend far beyond the ropes into the very fabric of my everyday life.

Through years of practice, I have come to understand that Shibari is not merely about bondage; it is about liberation. It is about creating a safe space where two people can explore the depths of their connection, where trust is both given and received. It is about the beauty of imperfection and the art of letting go, embracing the moment as it is and allowing oneself to be vulnerable.

Shibari has become my meditation, a practice that grounds me and allows me to express my creativity in ways I never imagined possible. It is a journey of self-discovery and artistic exploration, a path that continues to challenge and inspire me. As I tie the ropes, I find a sense of peace and fulfillment, a reminder of the power of human connection and the beauty that lies in surrender.

In writing this book, I hope to share the transformative experience of Shibari with you. Whether you are a curious beginner or an experienced practitioner, I invite you to join me on this journey—to explore the art and philosophy of Shibari, learn its techniques and nuances, and discover the profound impact it can have on your life and relationships. Together, we will delve into the rich history and cultural significance of Shibari, uncovering the secrets of this ancient art form and embracing its possibilities.

Welcome to the world of Shibari, a place where the ropes become an extension of your soul, and the ties bind you not just to your partner but to a community of artists and explorers who celebrate the art of connection. Let us embark on this journey together, and may it be one of discovery, creativity, and profound personal growth.

CHAPTER 1

EXPLORING JAPANESE ROPE BONDAGE

Welcome to the Shibari guide, where you'll learn the essentials of Japanese rope bondage! Today, we'll cover its history, foundational techniques, and essential safety tips.

For me, the systematic repetition and precise structure of rope bondage are incredibly calming. As a rope top, no matter what else is happening in my life, I must be present and focused on the ties, the person I'm tying, and the overall tone of the encounter. I find satisfaction in the dynamic of the bottom relinquishing control while enjoying the experience.

For those being tied, or "bottoms," the experience can also be deeply soothing. Many describe feeling relaxed and blissful while in rope. One individual shared, "I enjoy relinquishing control to the top, allowing them to do as they wish and feeling their power as they tie.

The sensation, pain, and restriction feel exquisite." Another remarked, "I derive pleasure from surrendering power, enjoying the psychological aspect of being restrained, and the challenge of enduring discomfort. It's liberating to have someone else—or the rope—control my movement. It's a safe space where I don't need to make decisions or be in control. It's soothing and helps me stay present."

Engaging in rope bondage often creates an emotionally intimate space. It can range from rough and sexual to gentle and non-sexual or anywhere in between.

WHAT IS SHIBARI

Shibari, also known as kinbaku, is a form of Japanese rope bondage distinct from its Western counterpart. It uses non-stretchy natural fiber ropes, like jute or hemp, instead of softer cotton, silk, or polyester ropes. Shibari focuses on friction and wraps rather than knots, uses the rope doubled over at the bight (the midpoint), and emphasizes the aesthetic appeal of the ties.

Shibari creates intricate ties by building on foundational blocks and repeated patterns. Once you learn these basics and safety principles, you can often replicate ties you've seen elsewhere. In the rest of this series, you'll explore several of these building blocks.

Shibari evolved from Hojojutsu, a martial art from Japan's Edo period (1600 to mid-1800s). During this period, samurai used Hojojutsu to arrest and restrain prisoners. Prisoners were often tied in ropes to convey their class and crime before execution or imprisonment. Hojojutsu faded after the Edo period when the shogunate fell.

In Japan, Hojojutsu ties were adapted for BDSM, exploring physical restraint and emotional shame. This art of tight and often painful sexual or sensual tying became known as Shibari (decorative tying) or kinbaku (tight binding).

Shibari has recently gained popularity in BDSM communities worldwide. While non-Japanese individuals may not fully grasp the cultural context of shame associated with being tied, the complexity, efficiency, and beauty of the ties themselves have garnered appreciation. Many renowned Japanese performers and rope tops travel globally to perform and teach workshops.

However, as Shibari has spread, there has been some cultural appropriation or exoticism, such as

non-Japanese individuals wearing kimonos or tying only small Asian women. It's essential to practice these ties with respect and understanding of their origins and focus on personal experience.

Evolution from Kinbaku to Shibari

Shibari its historical roots in Kinbaku to its modern incarnation is a testament to its adaptability and cultural significance. Understanding this evolution helps illuminate the rich tapestry of tradition and innovation that characterizes ShibaShibariy.

Kinbaku: The Traditional Roots

Kinbaku, often translated as "tight binding," originated from Hojojutsu, a martial art technique used by samurai to restrain prisoners with rope. This method was highly functional, with an emphasis on quick, efficient tying to subdue and transport captives. Over time, these techniques evolved beyond their martial origins, influenced by Japan's artistic and cultural movements.

In the early 20th century, Kinbaku began to appear in Japanese art, literature, and theater, reflecting a growing fascination with the aesthetic and emotional potential of rope bondage. Artists and writers explored themes of power, beauty, and restraint, bringing Kinbaku into the realm of erotic art and performance. This shift marked the beginning of Kinbaku's transformation into a form of artistic expression, where the ropes were used to create intricate patterns and evoke robust emotional responses.

Shibari: The Artistic Transformation

As Kinbaku continued to evolve, it gradually became known as Shibarihasizing the art and aesthetics of rope bondage rather than its functional aspects. This transformation was fueled by a growing appreciation for the visual and emotional impact of the ropes, as well as an interest in exploring the psychological dynamics between the rigger and the model.

Shibari artists began to focus on the beauty of the human form, using ropes to highlight the body's natural curves and contours. The ties became more elaborate and creative, incorporating elements of symmetry and asymmetry, tension and release. This artistic approach elevated performance art, where the process of tying became a dance of connection and expression.

Today, Shibarie recognized worldwide as a distinct art form, and it is celebrated for its ability to transcend cultural boundaries and communicate universal themes of trust, vulnerability, and beauty. Its evolution from Kinbaku reflects a broader cultural shift towards appreciating the depth and complexity of human relationships and the ways in which art can illuminate our shared experiences.

The Art and Philosophy of Japanese Rope Bondage

At its core, Shibari is more than a series of knots and ties; it is an art form that embraces the complexity and nuance of human relationships. The ropes become a medium through which the rigger (the person tying) and the model (the person being tied) engage in a dialogue that transcends words. Every wrap and knot speaks of trust, vulnerability, and intimacy, creating a unique experience for both participants.

Shibari is often compared to a dance, where each movement is deliberate and graceful, and every interaction is infused with intention and care. Its aesthetic appeal lies in Shibariity to transform the human form into a living sculpture, highlighting the curves and lines of the body while inviting the viewer to appreciate its natural beauty.

Beyond its visual impact, Shibari is deeply philosophical. It challenges conventional notions of power and control, exploring themes of surrender and empowerment. The ropes create a paradoxical space where the model experiences freedom through restraint, a journey into self-discovery and liberation that can be both profound and transformative.

For many practitioners, Shibari is also a Shibarif meditation, a practice that cultivates mindfulness and presence. It requires the rigger to be attuned to the model's physical and emotional state, responding with sensitivity and empathy to their needs and desires.

SOME COMMON KNOTS & FRICTIONS

Bight

"Bight" typically refers to the midpoint of the rope when folded in half. However, note that a "bight" is really any full bend in the rope, so you can create a bight at any location in the rope

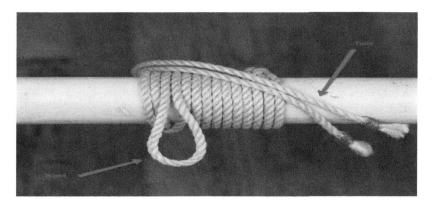

Lark's Head

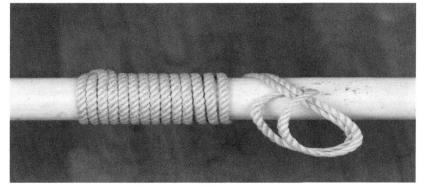

X-Friction

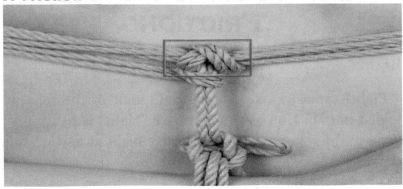

L-Friction

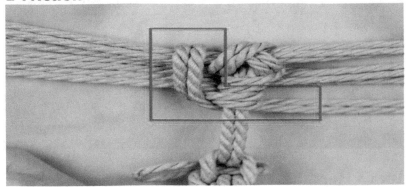

Half-Moon Friction

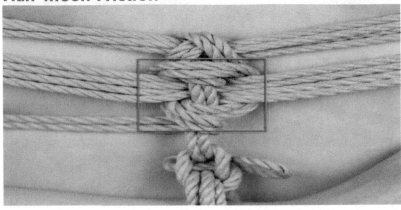

for extending rope

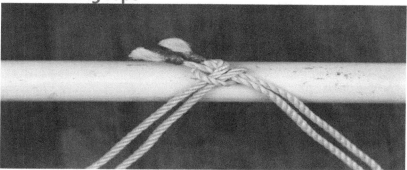

flipped lark's head

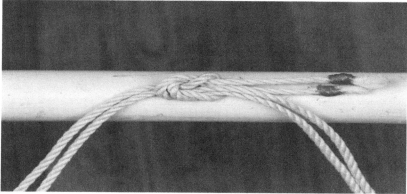

Reverse Tension

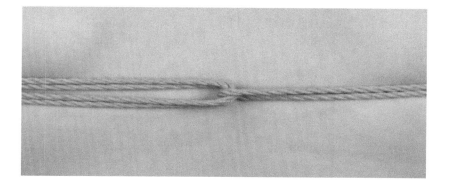

Cinch(kannuki)

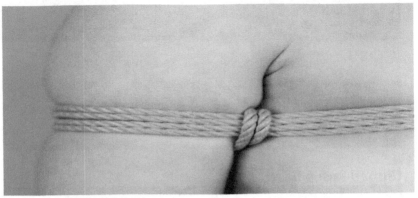

Inline Cuff / Hojo Cuff

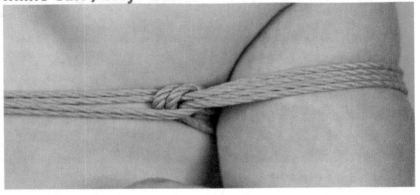

Friction (tomenawa) Turn / Direction Change

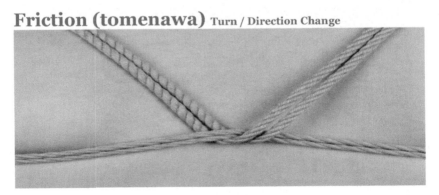

(nodome)

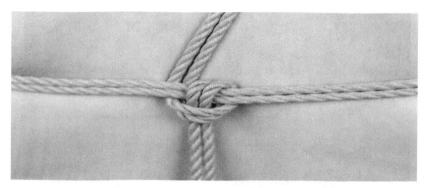

(uranodome)

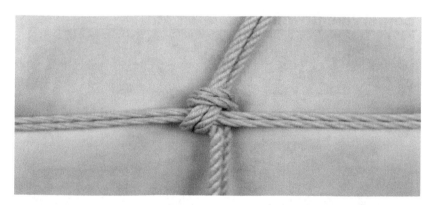

Upside-Down Munter

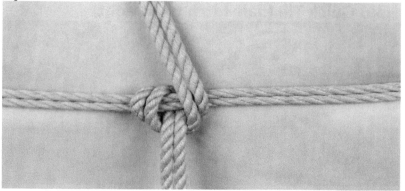

Square Knot

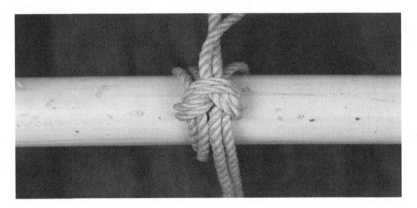

Somerville Bowline

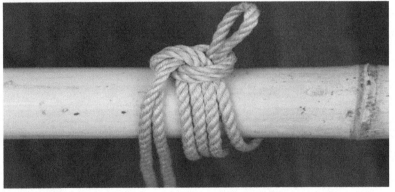

Hojo Quick Tie (half-hitch on a bight)

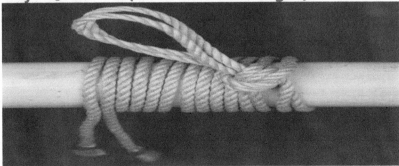

(Take dome)

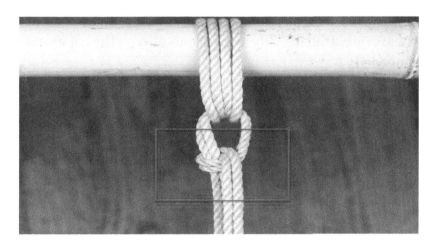

Understanding Consent and Safety

While Shibari is an art rooted in beauty and connection, it is also a practice that demands a deep understanding of consent and safety. The intimate nature of Shibari necessitates communication and mutual respect between all participants, ensuring that boundaries are respected and desires are honored.

Consent is the foundation of any Shibari session. Before the ropes even touch the skin, it is essential to engage in an open and honest dialogue about expectations, limits, and potential risks. This conversation should be ongoing, with both parties checking in regularly to ensure that the experience remains comfortable and consensual.

Safety is paramount in Shibari. The rope Shibarie beautiful, can pose risks if not handled with care and expertise. Understanding basic anatomy and being aware of sensitive areas such as nerves and circulation points is crucial to prevent injury. Practitioners must also be prepared to respond to any physical or emotional distress, with safety shears or cutters readily available to release the ropes quickly if needed.

Educating oneself through workshops, classes, and experienced mentors can provide valuable knowledge and skills, enhancing both safety and enjoyment. It is vital to approach Shibari with humiShibarid, a willingness to learn, acknowledging that mastery comes with time and practice.

Ultimately, Shibari is a jour exploration, one that invites participants to connect with themselves and each other in meaningful and transformative ways. By embracing the art and philosophy of Shibari while practicing consent and safety, one can experience the profound beauty and power of this ancient practice.

CHAPTER 2

CHOOSING YOUR ROPE

Jute and hemp are the most popular materials for shibari. The ropes are typically seven to eight meters long, four to six millimeters thick, and consist of three twisted strands. Natural fiber ropes are preferred because they provide grip, essential for shibari's wrapping techniques, which rely on friction rather than knots. They also look aesthetically pleasing and provide the tension desired by many bottoms.

Before use, jute and hemp ropes must be treated:

- Boiled to soften.

- Dried under tension to maintain shape.

- Singed with a flame to remove fuzz and oiled to prevent dryness.

You can either buy raw rope and treat it yourself or purchase pre-treated rope. I recommend buying pre-treated rope initially, but conditioning raw rope yourself can be rewarding later on.

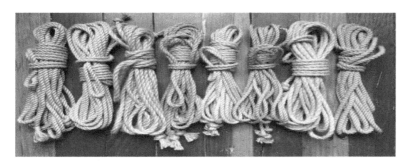

Image: Various shibari ropes, each 8m long and 6mm thick. From left to right: linen hemp (raw), jute (raw and stiff, needs treatment), jute (washed), jute (washed, roasted, and slippery), jute (tighter lay, soaked and roasted), hemp (raw, needs treatment), and synthetic.

Where to Buy Rope

- **Esinem Rope** (My favorite source and the only one offering linen hemp, which I love)

- **Jade Rope**

- **Twisted Monk**

- **Erin Houdini**

- **Kankinawa.com**

- **My Nawashi** (Etsy)

Caring for Natural Fiber Bondage Rope

The rope typically comes with a simple overhand knot at the ends to prevent fraying. You can keep these knots as is (and retie them when needed), whip the ends with waxed thread, or use a more complex knot. I've used a Sailmaker's Whipping with waxed sail thread on some of mine, and it has held up well with frequent use. Store rope in bundles (hanks) to avoid tangling and twisting.

Avoid washing your rope frequently. Washing, drying, singeing, and oiling weaken the fibers, making them unsafe for suspensions. It's best to keep your rope clean from the start. If you're planning crotch ties, set aside specific rope for that person or use synthetic rope, which can be machine-washed.

If your rope becomes dry, apply jojoba oil. Just rub a few drops in your palm and run the rope through your hands; don't overdo it.

Tying a Figure Eight Hank

To store the rope in a figure-eight hank, first gently straighten the rope to remove knots, kinks, or tension.

1. Grasp the two ends with your right hand. Move your left hand about 10 inches (25 cm) down the rope and create a loop with your thumb. Bring your left hand up and make another loop with your right thumb at the same distance down the rope. Alternate this motion until you have about 20 inches (50 cm) of rope remaining.

2. With about 20 inches (50 cm) left, tightly grasp the top of your rope bundle with your left hand.

3. Take the rope end and wrap it tightly around the bundle once. Wrap it again above the first wrap to lock it in place. Then, continue wrapping below the top wraps, keeping the rope taut.

4. On your final wrap, place your index and middle fingers over the wraps facing downward. Wrap the final loop over your fingers, bring it around, and grasp the rope between your fingers. Pull it through entirely or halfway to create a slip knot.

Untying a hank is quick, keeping your rope neat and tangle-free, with the bight ready to pull for untying.

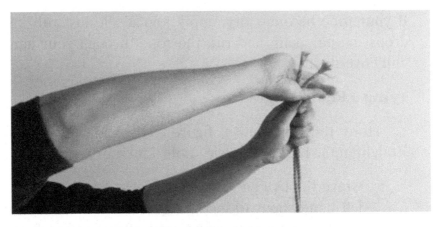

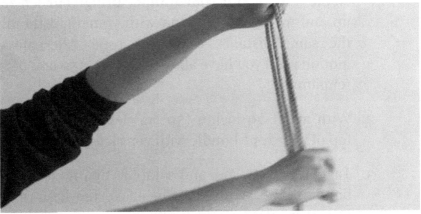

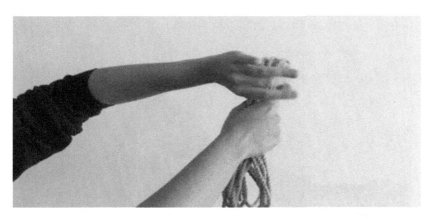

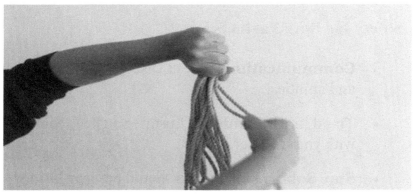

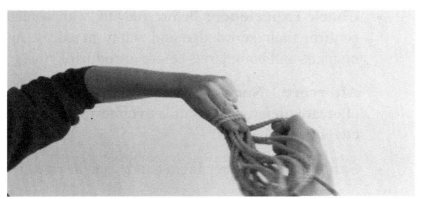

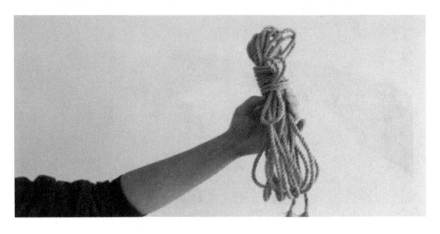

Safety for Both Partners

- **Communication is Key:** Discuss limits, experience, and abilities.

- **Trust and Comfort:** Ensure you feel comfortable with your partner.

- **Stay Sober:** Both parties should be clear-headed.

- **Check Experience:** Before playing with someone, confirm their knowledge and safety practices. Agree on plans and boundaries before introducing rope.

- **Aftercare Needs:** Discuss and communicate aftercare preferences (cuddles, comfort, snacks, space, etc.) before playing.

- **Safety Shears:** Keep them handy, just in case.

Safety Tips for Bottoms

- **Self-Check:** Ensure you're not claustrophobic or anxious about being in rope and are mentally prepared.

- **Disclose Injuries:** Inform your top of any physical injuries or conditions affecting flexibility or causing pain.

- **Pay Attention:** Notice any tingling, numbness, coldness, or burning in your limbs, especially your hands and fingers, and inform your top immediately. Silence can lead to severe, possibly permanent, nerve damage.

- **Speak Up:** If you need to be released from the rope, don't hesitate to tell your top.

Safety Tips for Tops Bottoms

- **Inquire About Injuries:** Ask if your bottom has any injuries or conditions affecting the ties.

- **Respect Boundaries:** Discuss body parts they want or don't want to be tied, touched, accentuated, or involved in the scene.

- **Monitor Physical Changes:** Before tying, check your bottom's hands for baseline color and temperature. If they change, adjust the ties. Ignoring these signs can lead to nerve damage.

- **Regular Check-ins:** Especially with new partners, ask how they're doing or establish non-verbal check-ins to maintain the mood.

- **Communication Methods:** Ensure your bottom has a way to communicate if gagged or unable to speak.

- **Stay Close:** Never leave your bottom alone for more than a couple of minutes, and always be within earshot.

- **Respond to Numbness:** If numbness occurs, remain calm, ask your bottom to move their extremities, and untie them if needed. Cut the rope if necessary.

- **Tie Over Muscle Groups:** Place ropes over large muscles like arms, thighs, chest, and hips.

- **Avoid Certain Areas:** Do not tie under the armpits or place knots on the back of the knee, inner wrists, or inner thighs. Beginners should avoid neckties.

- **Learn Basic Anatomy:** Understanding where muscles and nerves are located helps you tie safely.

- **Wrist Ties:** Hands often lose circulation first, so consider tying wrists last.

- **Quick Release:** If your bottom needs to be released, do so calmly and quickly. Reassure them and help with deep breathing. Cut the rope if necessary, as the rope can be replaced. Building trust is vital, so encourage open communication about limits for a better experience next time.

Single tie

Not only are single—and double-column ties entertaining on their own, but they also serve as the basis for many more intricate shibari ties. It is crucial to learn these two shibari knots, regardless of whether you want to use them alone or combine them into other designs. After you've mastered them, repeat the exercises until you can perform them without thinking.

Unblemished Shibari Tie

The most popular kind of shibari tie is a single-column tie. A column is anything you tie, such as a waist, a bedpost, a chair rung, or a leg. I'll provide an example of an arm below. Make sure you remove any watches or jewelry from your wrists before proceeding.

Locate the bight, or middle, of your rope first. Allow a space for a few fingers to slide between the rope and the wrist as you wrap it twice around the wrist (above the joint). Cross the working ends (the two rope ends that are opposite the bight) over the bight.

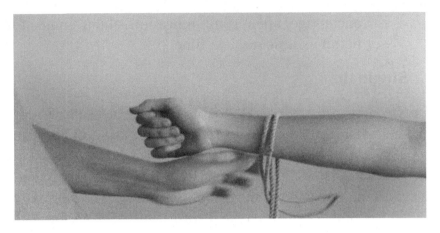

Slide the bight between all of the ropes. If you reach beneath it and pull it instead of pushing it through, the rope will always hold its lay (twist pattern) better and stay in shape.

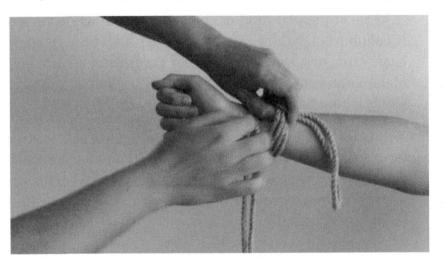

Using the working end, create a loop and draw the bight through. If, instead of forming a knot, the product comes apart, attempt to pull the bight through the other side.

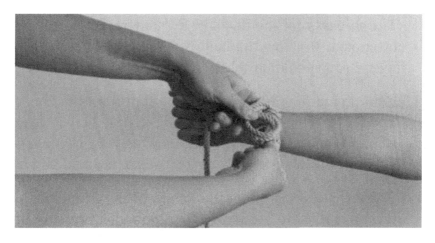

Make another loop and insert the bight once more. When you pull tightly on the knot, you should still be able to slide a few fingers between the ropes and your wrist; it shouldn't tighten at all on the wrist. And that's it!

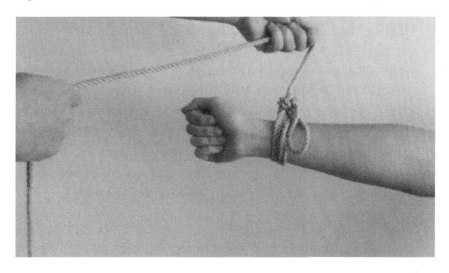

Remember

• The shibari knot should allow for some wrist movement but not enough to allow the hand to escape the tie. With a few fingers, you should be able to reach below the ropes.

• Some remaining braid loops should prevent the knot from unraveling. When you first start off, it's preferable to have a little bit longer remaining braid loop; as you get the hang of the knot, you can gradually make it seem neat and polished.

• The four ropes running the length of the wrist should not overlap or twist to avoid applying too much pressure in one area.

• To lessen the possibility of nerve injury, the knot is placed on the outside of the wrist rather than the delicate inner wrist and positioned a few inches above the hand.

Using the Bight as a Pulley

You may also employ the bight as a pulley system to safely fasten your bottom to anything else without putting undue strain on the ropes around your wrist, the knot, or your wrist itself. If you do tie your bottom over your partner's head, make sure it supports their own weight and doesn't dangle from their wrists, which might cause severe nerve damage. This is not a healthy technique for retaining weight.

First, wrap the ends of your rope around a bed post, a hard point (usually a hook or loop in the ceiling you can tie to), or anything else you can think of to use the bight as a pulley. Then, come back and thread the rope through the bight, then back through or around your point, and tie off all the ropes together in a double half hitch.

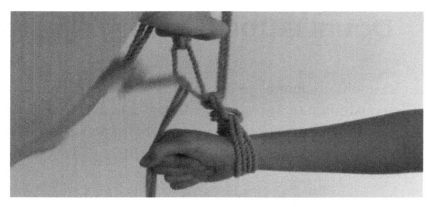

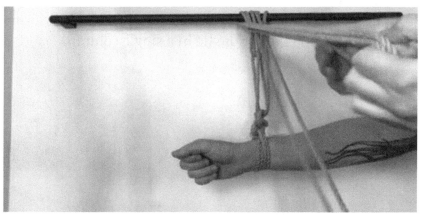

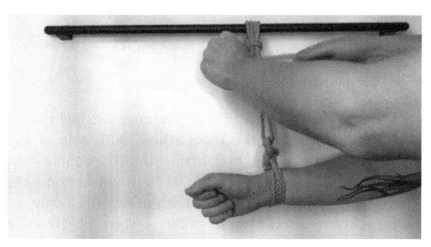

DOUBLE-COLUMN SHIBARI TIE

A double column joins two columns. While I'll be demonstrating on two wrists, you may also bind a wrist to a thigh, an ankle to a chair leg, an upper arm that is folded and cannot be utilized, or an ankle to an upper thigh with the knee bent.

Locate the middle or right of your rope first. Twist it twice around each wrist. Remember to give your bight a lot more slackly than you did for the tie in a single column.

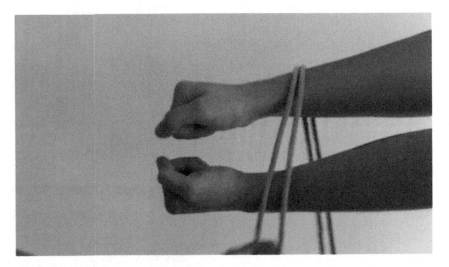

At the top and middle of the wrists, cross the bight over the working ends. Pass the rope behind both sets of ropes, through the wrists, and back to the front. The double-column tie wraps the bight over both the top and bottom sets of ropes, in contrast to the single-column tie, which only wraps the bight beneath the top set of ropes. The rope crosses both sets of ropes, passes between the two columns, and then rises back up.

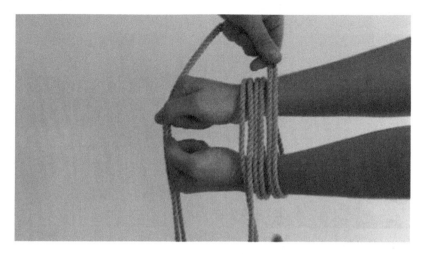

With the working end, create a loop and pull the bight through. If it merely breaks apart without forming a knot, try inserting the bight through the other side.

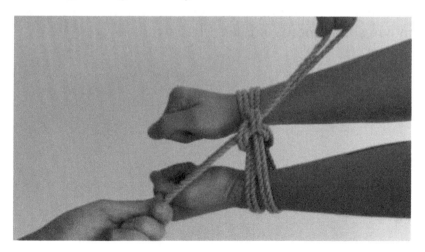

Make another loop and insert the bight once more. Pull firmly to lock the knots. You should be able to fit a few fingers between the ropes and the wrists without the knot being too loose to allow the hands to pass through, but it shouldn't tighten at all.

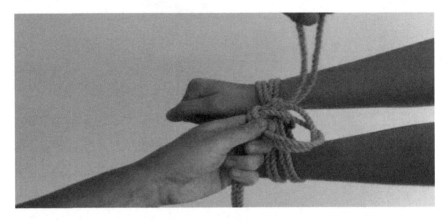

Practice, practice, and more practice!

Rehearse your single and double-column ties repeatedly on chair legs or your ankles until you can do them instinctively and without thinking. Mastering both is critical before moving on to more complex relationships.

SHIBARI LEG TIE

To begin a leg tie that will immobilize one leg, start by tying a single-column tie around the ankle. For a cleaner appearance, initiate the single-column tie by spiraling the bight down the ankle instead of up so the working ends are on top. After securing the single column, gently push the bottom's shin to bring the ankle as close to the lower thigh as possible. (This tie is delightful to practice on yourself, as it leaves most of your body and arms free.) It's essential to perform this step to prevent the ropes from becoming slack and loose as the bottom relaxes into the tie.

Next, spiral the working ends up the leg, ensuring that the first wrap is low on the thigh. Depending on the size of your bottom bottom's leg, you can make between two to four wraps (or more if you extend the rope). Start with three wraps as demonstrated, and if you find that you run out of rope before completing the tie, backtrack and try with two wraps. Conversely, if you have too much leftover rope, try using four wraps instead.

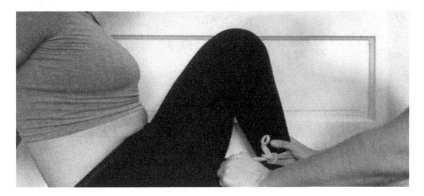

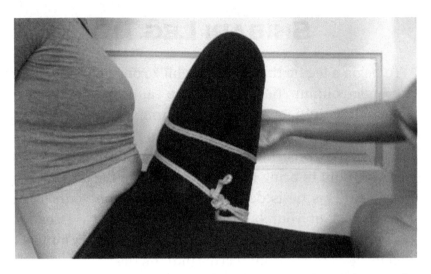

Pass the final rope of your spiral over itself on the inside of the knee, creating a small triangle. Insert your finger through this triangle, grab the rope, and pull it underneath. Use your other hand to pinch where the ropes cross to prevent them from sliding out of place. Next, take the working ends and bring them over the top rope, then under the left rope.

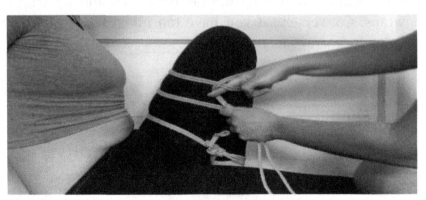

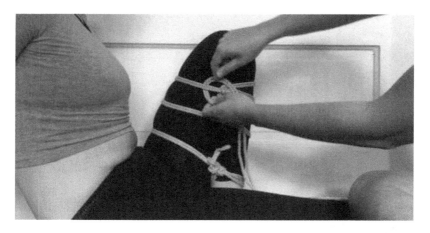

Repeat this knot on each rope, working down the spiral, including the bottom rope. Once you reach the end, pass the working ends through the leg and around to the other side.

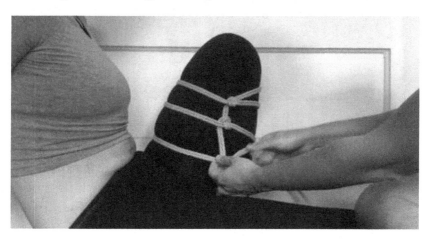

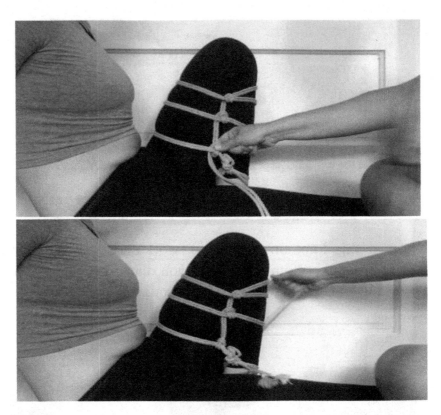

On the outside of the leg, pull the working ends to cinch the tie tightly. You will now repeat the knot on the outside of the leg, but in reverse, as the working ends are now moving upward instead of downward. Bring the working ends up over the bottom rope, back down on the right, then over the bottom rope again, and finally back up under the left rope.

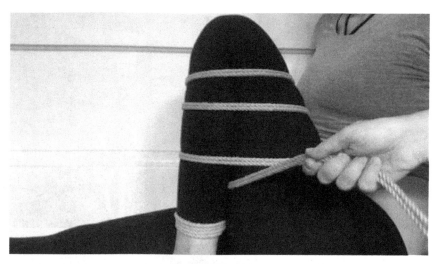

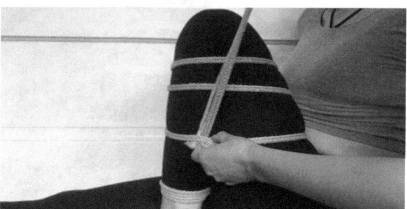

Repeat this step on each rope of the spiral until you reach the top.

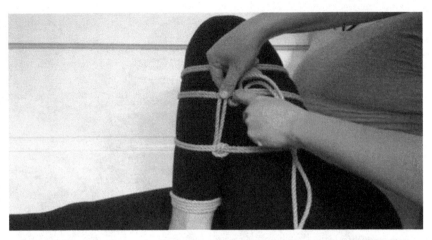

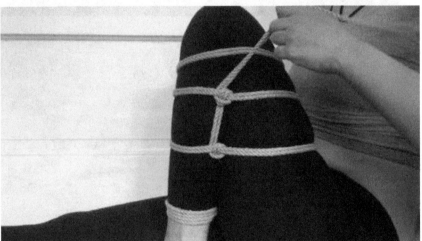

On the top rope's knot, finish by threading the working ends through the loop, reversing their direction so they go back down the leg again.

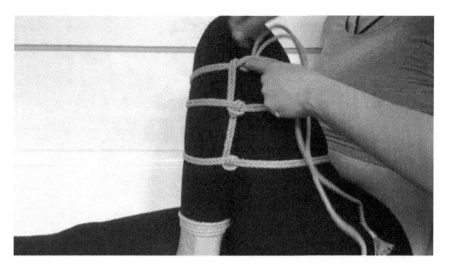

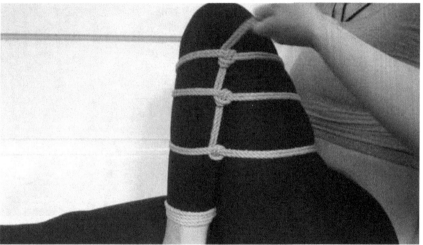

If you have leftover rope, twist it around the stem of the tie. Secure it with a hitch, and tuck the remaining rope around the stem or between the leg for a neat finish.

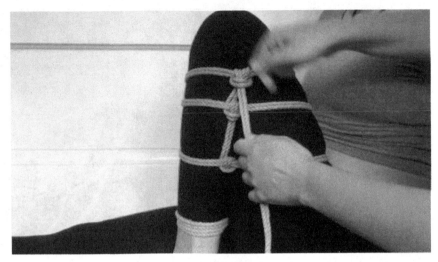

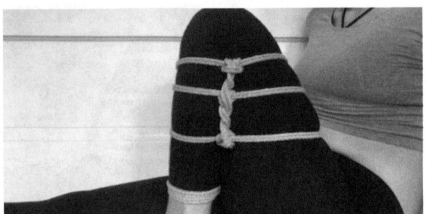

You're done

CHAPTER 3

SHIBARI HOGTIE

In this chapter, we're going to combine two ties we've learned before into a hogtie. A hogtie positions your bottom face down on the floor, secured by either a chest harness (which we've covered) or a box tie that includes the wrists. The ankles are then connected to the chest ties and pulled tightly. This method is safer than the Western-style hogtie, which ties the ankles to the wrists, as it distributes the weight of the legs across the chest instead of putting pressure on the sensitive wrists. You can opt for a simple double-column tie on the ankles or get more decorative by tying both legs using the leg tie we learned earlier.

1. **Tie the Chest Harness:** Begin by tying a chest harness on your bottom. When extending the rope, ensure that there are no knots on the sternum or other sensitive chest areas that might cause discomfort when your bottom lies chest-down.

2. **Position Your Bottom:** Lay your bottom on their belly. If you want to incorporate their arms, use a new rope or the leftover rope from the chest harness to tie a single-column tie around the wrists. Ensure the inside of their wrists are touching to protect the sensitive inner wrists. Then, apply a double-column tie to their ankles.

3. **Connect the Ties:** Take the ends of the ankle ropes and pass them through the center column (spine) of

the chest harness. Make sure to go over and not include the ropes used to tie the wrists (if tied), ensuring that no pressure is applied to the wrist tie.

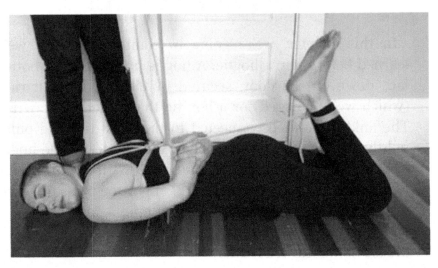

Then, loop the rope through the bight at the ankle, and bring it back through the center column (spine) of the chest harness again.

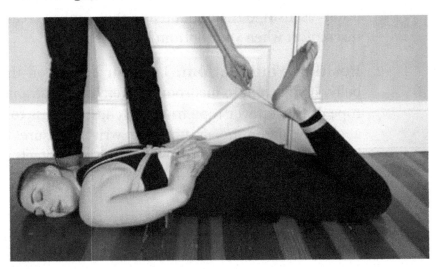

Tighten the tie until it is snug, ensuring that your bottom is not overextended or uncomfortable. Secure the rope with a half hitch to finish.

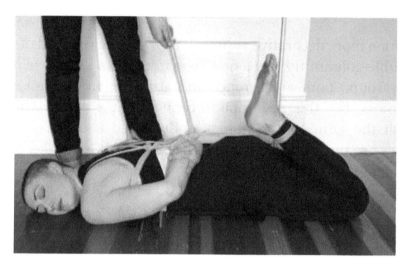

Tighten the tie until it is snug, ensuring that your bottom is not overextended or uncomfortable. Secure the rope with a half hitch, and then add another half hitch to ensure it is firmly tied.

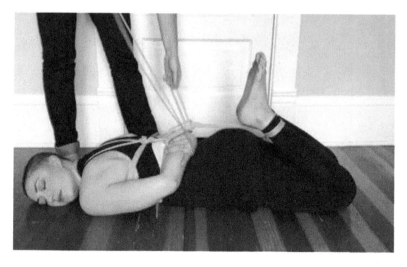

If the rope places too much pressure on the wrists, consider tying it around the top of the chest harness instead. Pass the ropes behind both shoulder ropes, right above the top knot, and secure them in the same way.

For a more decorative approach using leg ties instead of the double-column tie, use a new rope to create a single-column tie around both ankle ropes and attach them to the chest harness. Use this new rope to connect to the chest harness with the same pulley system as described above. You can even use two different ropes to tie the ankles apart, keeping the legs separated instead of bound together.

How To Tie your partner HAND

Tying people up can be fun! But how do you do it safely and consensually? Whether you're tying up your girlfriend or another activity partner, it's essential to know how to proceed for the first time.

Communication is Key

Before engaging in any bondage, have an open conversation with your activity partner about preferences and boundaries. Discuss what you both enjoy, what you want to try, what you might be open to trying, and what is off-limits. Creating a yes/no/maybe list can be helpful. If neither of you has experience with bondage, it's normal not to know how you'll react or feel, so take it slow and check in frequently.

If your play involves one partner saying "no" or "stop" and another ignoring it, establish a transparent verbal or physical signaling system that's out of context, such as using stoplight colors or dropping something small and loud. The goal is to have fun while keeping it safe, sane, and consensual, and communication is a vital part of that.

Choosing the Right Rope

For bondage, thick silk rope is excellent as it only slides or moves a little once secured. Hemp and jute are perfect for shibari. However, these options can be expensive. If you're not ready to invest heavily, consider using solid-braid nylon rope, 1/4" to 7/16" in diameter, available at hardware stores or online. This type of rope maintains knots that are easy to untie, even under tension.

In earlier versions of this guide, thick cotton rope was recommended due to its availability, affordability, and machine washability. However, cotton constricts when wet (e.g., from sweat), so consider alternatives first. Rope is versatile and can be used for handcuffs, floggers, strap-on harnesses, belts, and countless restraint methods.

Safety Tips

Before you start tying, keep these safety tips in mind:

- **Looseness:** Keep the rope loose enough to slide two fingers between the rope and your partner's skin. The goal is to restrain, not cut off, circulation. If the rope might get wet (such as when using cotton rope), leave it even looser.

- **Circulation Checks:** Monitor circulation by watching for skin that turns blue or white. Check-in with your partner often, and ensure they alert you to any pins and needles or numbness.

- **Breathing:** Never tie the rope in a way that restricts breathing.

- **Supervision:** Never leave someone tied up alone.

- **Safety Scissors:** Keep blunt-edged medical safety scissors nearby in case you need to release someone quickly.

- **Take It Slow:** Don't rush. If you feel self-conscious about going slowly, try tying your partner's hands behind their Back. They won't see what you're doing, allowing you to check instructions discreetly. Moving slowly can also enhance the experience. To boost confidence, consider blindfolding them.

Creating Rope Handcuffs

These instructions are inspired by *Back on the Ropes* by Two Knotty Boys, a step-by-step guide to rope bondage. While the directions below focus on tying wrists together, you can apply the same technique to ankles, wrists to ankles, or tying to furniture. The wrap is thick enough to feel solid and comfortable. You can leave ropes dangling to guide your partner or tuck them in to lead them by the wrap.

You Will Need:

- 25 feet of rope

- A willing partner (or an upside-down chair for practice)

- Blunt-edged scissors (just in case)

Directions:

1. **Position:** Have your partner hold their wrists out with about two fists of space between them. Lay the rope over their wrists so that the middle of the rope is roughly between their hands.

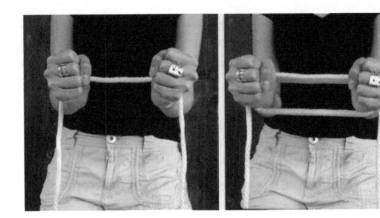

2, Wrap: Wrap each end around the wrists twice for a total of five wraps.

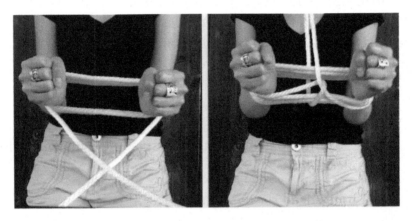

3, Continue Wrapping: Wrap each end of the rope around, moving towards your partner's wrists. Stop wrapping when there is still a small gap between the wrapped rope and their skin. Aim for an equal number of wraps on each side of the first crossed ropes. If the wraps appear loose, twist each side in the direction you wound it to tighten everything. You may need to wrap each end once or twice more to ensure a secure fit.

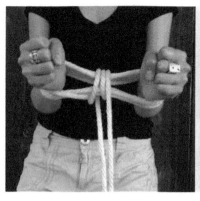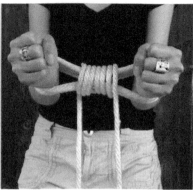

4. Secure the Wrap: Lift the last loop on the left side and tuck the end of the rope through the resulting circle from the inside to the outside. Repeat this on the other side to tie everything off. Pull on both ends of the rope to secure it tightly. You can either tuck the remaining ends into the wrap if they're short or use them to tie your partner to something else.

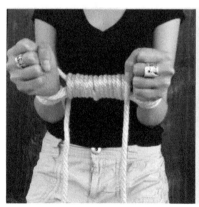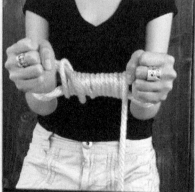

Congratulations, you've successfully tied someone up!

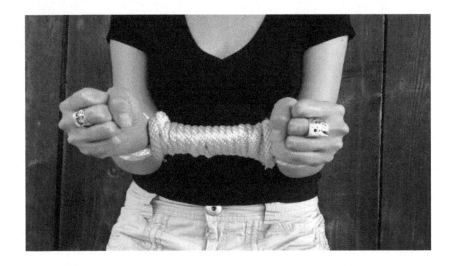

SHIBARI CHEST HARNESS

In Shibari, a chest harness can serve as a standalone tie or as a foundation for securing other ties. This version is simple, but once you master it, you can create more intricate and decorative variations.

Position the Bight: Start by placing the bight (the midpoint of the rope) at the center of your bottom's back.

Wrap the Rope: Wrap the rope once around your bottom's body, positioning it below the chest. Pull the working ends through the bight.

Adjust the Cross: Ensure the part where the rope crosses over is aligned with the middle of the back, directly on the spine.

Check Tightness: The ropes should be snug but not so tight that they restrict your bottom's ability to breathe.

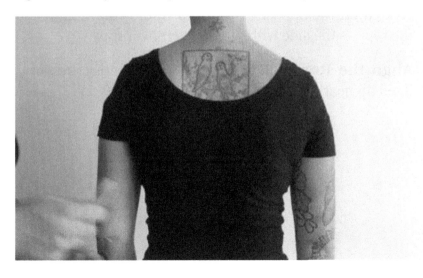

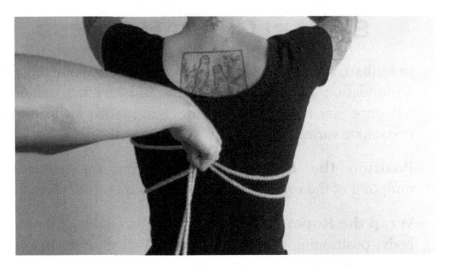

Wrap Around Again: Bring the working ends back around the front of the body in the opposite direction. This change in direction is crucial to ensure the rope stays tight and doesn't slip off the body.

Secure at the Back: When you reach the center of the back again, pull the working ends up through the loop you just created on the opposite side from where you initially pulled the rope — the side with the doubled-over rope.

Align the Ropes: Ensure the ropes do not cross and are lined up neatly for a clean appearance.

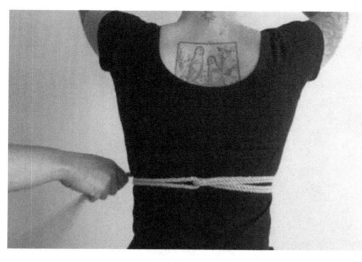

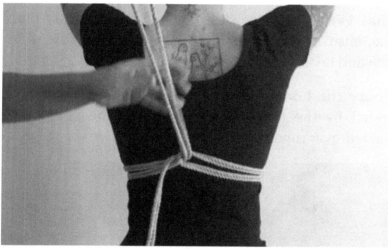

Reverse Direction: Change direction once more and bring the working ends around the body again, this time positioning them above the chest.

Secure the Rope Stem: Wrap the working ends underneath the rope stem, which is the vertical section of rope running along the spine.

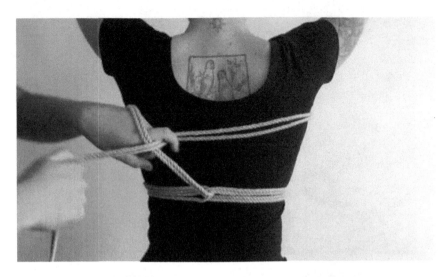

Final Wrap: Reverse direction around the body one last time, ensuring the ropes are positioned above the previous wrap and lie flat and neat.

Secure the Loop: Bring the working ends through the loop created by the change in direction — the side with the doubled-over rope.

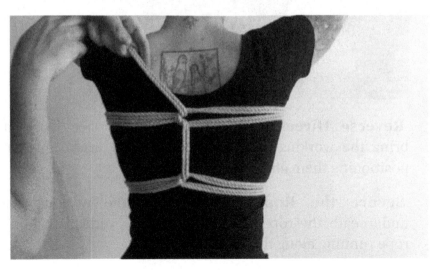

Bring the Ropes Over the Shoulder: Take the working ends and bring them over the shoulders to the front of your bottom.

Weave Through the Front Ropes: Pass the working ends over the top ropes in front and then under the bottom ropes. Pinch the bottom ropes together to maintain their shape as you reverse the direction with the working ends.

Reverse Direction: Bring the working ends back up and under the second set of top ropes.

Adjust the Knot: Ensure the knot is in a comfortable position for your bottom. If needed, adjust the knot slightly down the first rope to improve comfort.

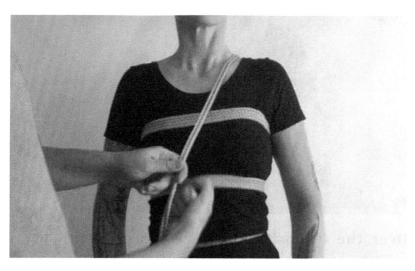

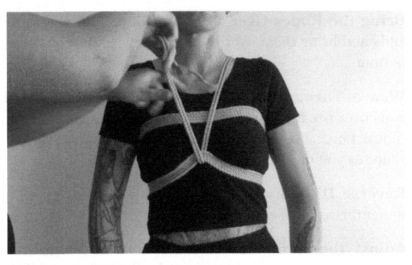

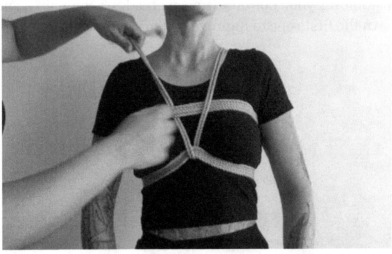

Over the Opposite Shoulder: Bring the working ends over the opposite shoulder and around to the back of your bottom.

Secure at the Back: Pass the working ends over the top proper ropes and then weave them up diagonally between the top left ropes and the left shoulder rope, as shown.

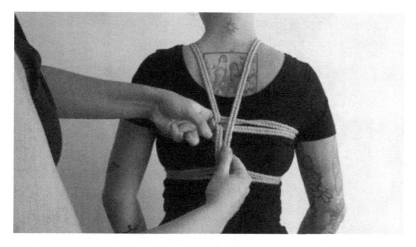

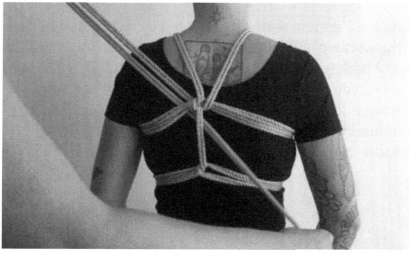

Bring the working ends over both shoulder ropes, and under the right top ropes.

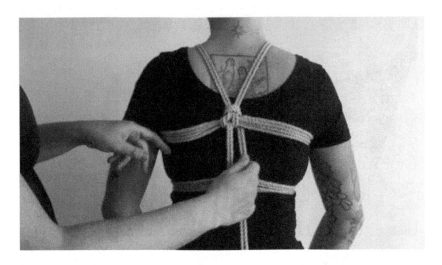

Attach the stem with a half hitch. To create a half hitch, loop the working ends together, then pass the ropes over, behind, and back through the loop. To tighten, pull. If you have extra rope, you may tie it to a hard point (not for suspension), leave it long to connect to an extra arm or leg tie, or wrap it around the stem and/or weave it up the shoulder ropes in a figure-eight weave.

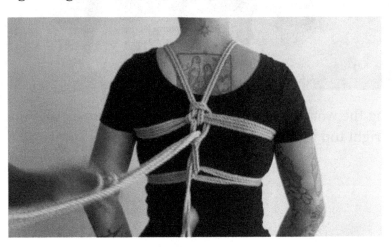

You've successfully constructed a simple shibari chest harness!

Stretching the Shibari Rope

When you run out of rope, you'll have to stretch it. There are several methods to do this.

Grasping the ropes with your other hand, reach inside the bight, draw the bight over your hand, and create a loop with your second rope. There will be a loop on your head, often known as a lark's head knot.

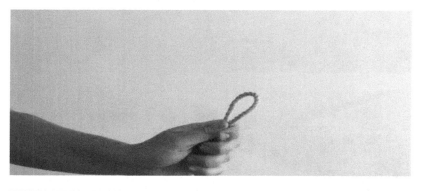

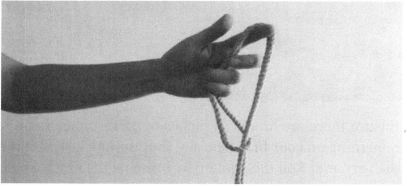

Tighten after inserting the ends of the first rope into the lark's head. You may carry the lark's head knot down to the knots and stop here if the ends of your ropes are knotted. Proceed to the next stage if you feel like it or if you have whipped ends.

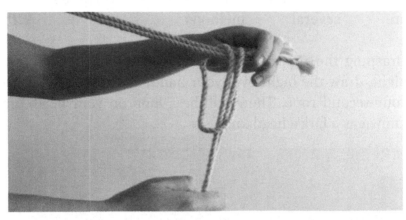

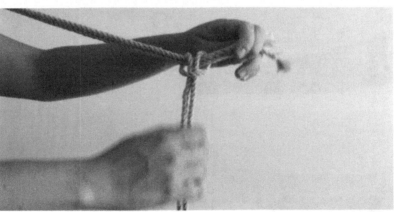

Ensure there are around 5 inches or 12 centimeters of ends remaining on your first rope and that the lark's head is not at the very end. Roll the knot up by bringing the first rope's two sides together.

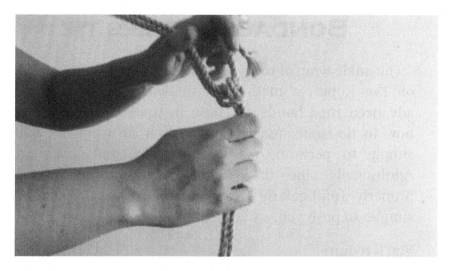

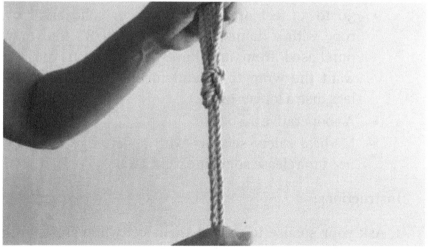

And that's it!

BONDAGE ANKLES TIE

The ankle wrap of today is based on Two Knotty Boys' Back on the Ropes, a methodical manual for both basic and advanced rope bondage. These instructions will show you how to tie someone's ankles together in a method that is simple to perform, feels comfortable, and looks great. Additionally, since they are unable to stand or even hop properly (particularly when wearing boots), it makes it simpler to push your exercise partner about.

You'll require:

- 30 to 55 feet of bondage rope or solid-braid nylon rope with a diameter of 7/16″ or 3/8″ that may be purchased from any hardware shop. If you would want the wrap to extend further up your partner's legs, use a longer piece.)
- A cooperative associate
- Medical safety scissors with a flat edge in case you need to release someone right away

Instructions:

1. Ask your spouse to stretch their feet while crossing their ankles slightly. To make a bright, find the center of the rope and fold it in half.

2. Bring the right over and under to the arch of their lower foot while holding the rope's working ends over the top of their ankles.

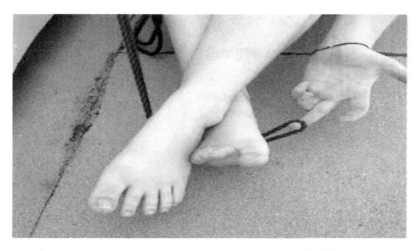

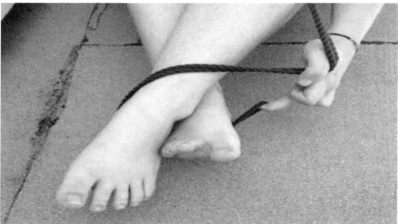

3. Keeping the bight in place, loop the rope's working ends over the front and down the back of both ankles.

4. Thread the working end through the narrow opening.

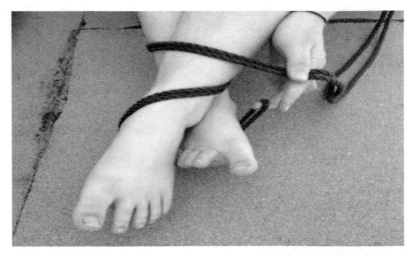

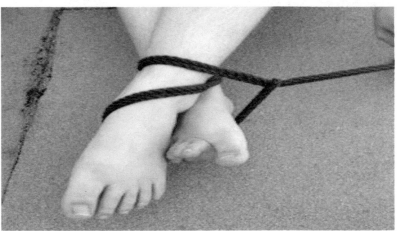

5. Reverse the direction of the working end and bring it up and over your partner's ankles while maintaining the ropes parallel to the ones that are already in place. While working, keep the ropes taut at all times.

6. To ensure that they are level and in line with the existing ropes, wrap the working end around behind their ankles. After that, they continue wrapping up their legs and around their ankles.

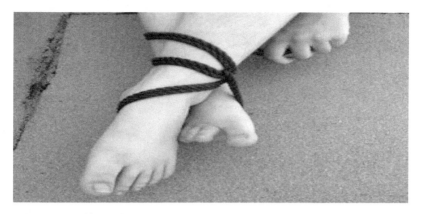

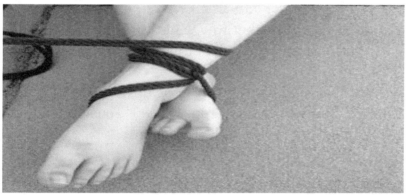

7. Continue wrapping!

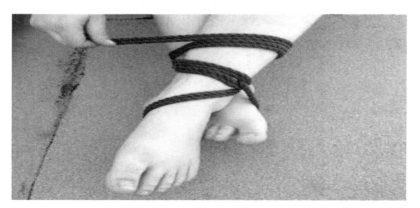

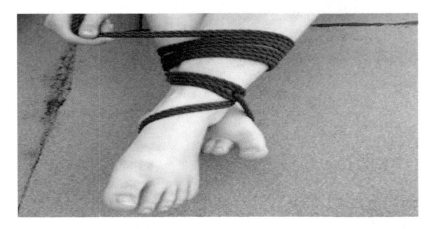

8. Double back the other way while holding the rope in place with your finger when it's time to knot everything off.

9. After that, pull the working ends through the loop and up through the uppermost rope layer. Tension should be maintained, but leave a little loop open.

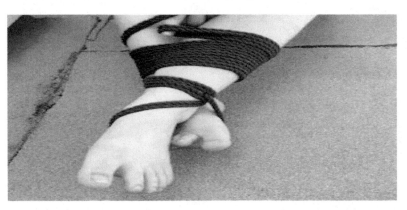

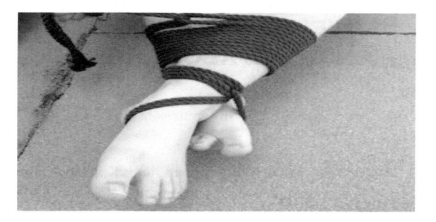

10. Tighten after passing the working ends through this loop.

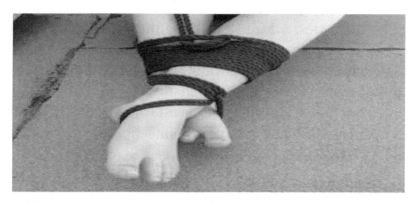

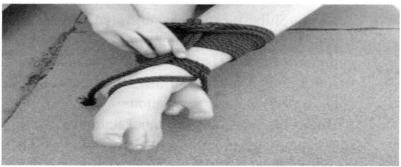

Well done, you've tied someone up!

SIGNIFICANT QUESTIONS AND ANSWERS ABOUT SHIBARI

Question: What is the difference between Shibari and Kinbaku?

- Answer: While both Shibari and Kinbaku refer to Japanese rope bondage, they have slightly different connotations. Shibari, which means "to tie" or "to bind," emphasizes the artistic and aesthetic aspects of rope bondage, focusing on the beauty and creativity of the ties. Kinbaku, meaning "tight binding," historically refers to the functional use of ropes in martial arts and restraint. Over time, the terms have become somewhat interchangeable in modern usage, but Shibari is often associated with artistic expression, while Kinbaku retains a connection to its traditional roots.

Question: Is Shibari safe?

- Answer: Shibari can be safe when practiced with proper knowledge, attention to detail, and communication. Safety is paramount, and practitioners must prioritize consent, open communication, and continuous awareness of their partner's physical and emotional state. It's essential to understand basic anatomy, avoid pressure points, and regularly check for signs of discomfort or circulation issues. Always have safety shears or cutters on hand to quickly release the ropes if needed. Educating yourself through workshops, classes, and resources can significantly enhance the safety of your practice.

Question: How do I start learning Shibari?

- Answer: The best way to start learning Shibari is by attending workshops or classes led by experienced practitioners. These settings provide hands-on instruction, guidance, and the opportunity to ask questions in a safe environment. Online tutorials and books, such as this one, can also offer valuable information for self-study. Begin with the basics, focusing on mastering knots and simple ties before progressing to more complex patterns and techniques. Practice regularly, prioritize safety, and engage with the Shibari community to deepen your understanding and skills.

Question: What type of rope should I use for Shibari?

- Answer: The choice of rope depends on personal preference and the intended use. Natural fiber ropes like jute and hemp are popular choices for Shibari due to their strength, grip, and traditional aesthetic. Jute is lightweight and has a slightly rough texture, while hemp is heavier and softer. Cotton ropes are gentle on the skin and ideal for beginners. Synthetic ropes like nylon and polyester are smooth and easy to clean but may require more attention to securing knots. Consider the diameter of the rope, with standard sizes ranging from 5mm to 8mm, depending on the desired level of support and precision.

Question: Can Shibari be practiced solo?

- Answer: Yes, Shibari can be practiced solo, often referred to as self-tying or self-suspension. Solo practice allows individuals to explore the art form independently, experimenting with patterns and techniques on their bodies. It can be a meditative and creative experience, offering a different perspective on Shibari. However, solo practitioners must be especially vigilant about safety, ensuring they can quickly release themselves if necessary and avoiding positions that could pose a risk if left unattended. Proper planning and preparation are essential for safe solo practice.

Question: How do I communicate with my partner about Shibari?

Answer: Effective communication is crucial in Shibari. Before beginning any session:

1. Have an open and honest conversation with your partner about expectations, boundaries, and desires.

2. Discuss any specific concerns or limitations, and establish a safe word or signal to indicate when something needs to change.

3. Throughout the session, maintain regular check-ins to ensure comfort and consent.

Active listening and empathy are vital to building trust and creating a positive experience for both parties.

Question: Is Shibari only for couples?

- Answer: While Shibari is often practiced between couples, it is not exclusive to romantic relationships. Shibari can be a shared experience between friends and collaborators or within a community setting, where trust and communication are prioritized. It can also be practiced as a form of artistic expression, performance, or self-exploration, allowing individuals to connect with themselves and others in unique ways. The key is to approach Shibari with respect, consent, and a shared understanding of the intentions and boundaries involved.

Question how can Shibari enhance intimacy?

- Answer: Shibari can enhance intimacy by fostering trust, communication, and vulnerability between partners. The process of tying and being tied requires collaboration, attention, and presence, creating a space where both parties can connect on a deeper level. Shibari encourages participants to explore their desires, boundaries, and emotions, allowing them to express themselves and understand each other in new and meaningful ways. The shared experience of Shibari can strengthen the bond between partners, offering a unique form of intimacy that extends beyond physical touch.

CONCLUSION

As we reach the end of our exploration into the world of Shibari, I invite you to reflect on the journey you've undertaken and the discoveries you've made along the way. Shibari is a multifaceted art form rich in history, creativity, and emotion. It is a practice that transcends the physical act of tying, inviting us to connect deeply with ourselves and others through trust, vulnerability, and expression.

Throughout this book, we've delved into the essential techniques and philosophies that form the foundation of Shibari. From the intricate knots and ties to the creation of beautiful harnesses, you've learned to harness the power of rope to craft experiences that are both visually stunning and emotionally resonant. But beyond the techniques, Shibari is about the connections we forge and the stories we tell through the dance of rope and body.

For many, Shibari serves as a path to self-discovery, a journey into the depths of our desires and emotions. It challenges us to confront our vulnerabilities and embrace the unknown, offering a space where we can explore our boundaries and push the limits of our creativity. It is a journey that is as personal as it is shared, inviting us to communicate openly and honestly with our partners and us.

As you continue your practice, remember that Shibari is an ever-evolving art form, one that encourages experimentation, innovation, and growth. Embrace the opportunity to learn from others, whether through workshops, community events, or collaborative projects.

Each interaction, each session, is a chance to deepen your understanding and expand your skill set.

Let Shibari be a source of inspiration, a reminder of the beauty that lies in connection and creativity. Allow it to challenge you, to surprise you, and to bring joy and fulfillment to your life. Whether you practice Shibari as an artistic expression, a form of intimacy, or a path to self-discovery, may it continue to enrich your journey and reveal new dimensions of yourself and those you share it with.

As you tie the final knot, remember that this is just the beginning. The world of Shibari is vast and varied, with endless possibilities for exploration and growth. Continue to pursue your passion with curiosity and enthusiasm, and let the ropes guide you to new and exciting experiences.

Thank you for embarking on this journey with me. May your exploration of Shibari bring you joy, connection, and a deeper understanding of the art of tying

Made in the USA
Coppell, TX
07 October 2024

38276313R00046